Shocking Medical Coverups

Proven solutions for beating diabetes, cancer, Alzheimer's, arthritis and more…

By Matthew Simons

All material in this publication is provided for information only and may not be construed as medical advice or instruction. No action or inaction should be taken based solely on the contents of this publication; instead, readers should consult appropriate health professionals on any matter relating to their health and well-being. This information and opinions provided in this publication are believed to be accurate and sound, based on the best judgment available to the authors. Readers who fail to consult with appropriate health authorities assume the risk of any injuries.

TABLE OF CONTENTS

A gang of terrorists attacked the clinic...

It wasn't even 9 am.

The doors to Dr. Jonathan V. Wright's clinic were still locked. One patient was waiting quietly in her wheelchair outside.

There was no warning of the violence about to happen.

Suddenly, a convoy of vehicles sped into the parking lot and two dozen heavily armed thugs got out.

With gun drawn, one of them kicked down the door to the clinic and barged inside...with more pistol-packing henchmen right behind.

One of them stuck a revolver in the receptionist's face. A female staff member who tried to call for help was thrown roughly in a chair and the phone lines ripped out of the wall.

The gang of thugs actually held the staff at gun point for 2 hours, then kicked them out of the building. They ransacked the clinic, destroyed medical equipment and pawed through confidential patient records.

It was like some terrorist nightmare out of Afghanistan or Kosovo. But the truth was even scarier...

The terrorists were wearing GOVERNMENT BADGES

They were sent to harass Dr. Wright by the FDA. And what was his "offense?" Was he selling drugs illegally? Giving out phony prescriptions over the Internet? Oh no... He was using preservative-free B vitamins. That's it. B VITAMINS.

Of course, no charges were ever filed. Even two Federal grand juries didn't return an indictment. Nope, the government heavies were just trying to send Dr. Wright a message, but, frankly, they should have picked an easier target to bully...

Because no other doctor in the world has worked harder, risked more and produced more truly brilliant natural solutions to the medical problems that threaten us most. And he won't let anything get in the way of his work.

Especially when the need for his 'miracle medicine' has now become *urgent*...

As dozens of best selling drugs bite the dust...now what?

Ever wondered, "Where do we go from here"?

One Doctor Who's Saving Modern Medicine

Natural Medicine's *LIFETIME ACHIEVEMENT AWARD* is just the latest in a long list of honors bestowed upon Jonathan V. Wright, MD by fellow doctors. He's President Emeritus of the National Health Federation and has served on the Board of Directors of Bastyr University, The Life Extension Foundation, the American Association for Health Freedom and other important institutions. And lately he's been appointed Trustee of prestigious Harborview Hospital in Seattle.

He has degrees from Harvard University (cum laude) and the University of Michigan, but unlike some "gurus" he doesn't like or need to trumpet his academic credentials. In fact, I had to cajole him to even allow me to write about his extraordinarily impressive accomplishments. But the truth is, his characteristic modesty does

Millions of people in pain are feeling betrayed by the recent Vioxx crisis, but as you'll see, *it's far from over*.

Dozens more drugs your loved ones depend on will make the headlines next.

nothing to diminish his fame...

Because his medical breakthroughs speak for themselves. He's the doctor who introduced bio-identical hormone replacement therapy for women. Developed the first successful treatment to reverse macular degeneration.

And he introduced Americans to the entire concept of natural medicine with articles in "Let's Live"...and introduced doctors to it in his best selling Book of Nutritional Therapy and Guide to Healing with Nutrition, as well as other classics in the field...

More than 3000 doctors, nurses and other health professionals have taken the famous seminars taught by Dr. Wright and his colleague, Alan Gaby, MD, acclaimed as the #1 educational resource for physicians who want to learn nutritional medicine...

Yet for Dr. Wright, all of the above is secondary to his family medical practice. At his world-acclaimed Tahoma Clinic, he's received over 38,000 patient visits from people who have come from as far away as Brazil, France, Japan and Thailand.

Squeezed for profit, *drug firms are rushing products to market before they're ready...*

New cholesterol drugs that may weaken the heart...

New prostate drugs suspected of encouraging cancer...

Cox-2 painkillers now linked to sudden death...

And in many cases, they don't even suppress the symptoms they're supposed to!

Has drug development hit a dead end? Could this once mighty pipeline be running dry? Even stock market analysts are saying it, but...

Dr. Jonathan V. Wright is leading the way to an AMAZING NEW KIND OF MEDICINE

Decades ago, Dr. Wright insisted that deadly side-effects were built into the entire system of drug development. The biggest profits come from patented drugs — and to get patents, you have to "improve" on nature. Yet, in a brilliant flash of insight, Dr. Wright saw this endeavor was doomed.

Because you can't possibly make a failing

body as good as new, unless you use "parts" identical to nature.

"Would you fix a Ford with Buick parts?" he asked. "*Of course not!*"

Our "replacement parts" must by identical to nature's original equipment.

Or else you're courting a lifetime of breakdowns. So Dr. Wright set out to create a therapy that works with nature, instead of against it. At the first, mainstream authorities ridiculed the very idea…

Some said, "Cure cancer with eggplant? *Impossible!*" But Dr. Wright published the research that showed success in 80,000 cases with zero cases of cancer return. (You can read all about it in Chapter Three.)

Others exclaimed, "Treat diabetes with cinnamon? *Preposterous!*" But then Dr. Wright uncovered research that demonstrated cinnamon's *near-miraculous effects* — and how it can also prevent diabetes from ever threatening your loved ones. (It's waiting for you in Chapter Two.)

In much the same way, he's helped tens of thousands of patients heal themselves of conditions from chronic infections to heart disease…using nothing more complicated than remedies like iodide and sugar cane.

Now thousands of forward-thinking doctors have flocked to his cause

They're calling him one of the greatest geniuses in contemporary medicine. And recently, fellow physicians paid him the ultimate tribute, honoring him with the very first *Linus Pauling Award* for Lifetime Achievement in Natural Medicine.

In this book, you'll learn about a few of the breakthroughs that deliver what drugs only promise…discoveries that out-distance the wildest dreams of drug research. In decades to come, they'll totally change what doctors can do for you.

But I don't want you to wait. *You deserve to have these revelations today.* Keep reading…

CHAPTER ONE

The 26-cent miracle that knocks out Alzheimer's

Is it possible that a so-called "crazy person's" mineral could be the hidden key to abolishing Alzheimer's?

Yes — and it's effective, 20 times cheaper and far safer than any prescription drug...

It's true. Those suffering from what scientists call "The Plague of the 21st Century" — can take heart, because, thanks to Dr. Wright, *there is hope*...

And it's coming in the form of an unlikely mineral straight from Mother Nature. It's astounding scientists and proving Alzheimer's is NOT a death sentence and it doesn't have to mean losing your independence, your dignity or your freedom.

Quite frankly, mainstream medicine is stumped when it comes to Alzheimer's

They don't understand why it strikes, how it erodes your mind, or how to get rid of it once it does.

The only thing they DO understand is how to overcharge you for useless pills...and how to recommend a good nursing home.

But no matter what you've heard, just know that you DON'T have to lose your wits to this dreaded disease. Natural treatments exist — and fortunately for you, they're much cheaper and often more effective than anything requiring a prescription.

Keep your memory, wit and independence…as this miracle mineral may actually rebuild your brain

Dr. Wright believes a landmark study has confirmed what scientists once thought impossible...that you can actually "regrow" and regenerate your brain — at any age.

This led the main researcher to exclaim: "This is the first demonstration of a pharmacological (drug) increase of human brain matter."

So what is this mineral miracle that's been hiding under our noses the whole time?

It's...lithium.

Now bear with me here. Most people think lithium's for loons in straight-jackets. But that's *lithium carbonate* — which is only available with a prescription and used to treat bipolar disorder. Truth be told, lithium isn't a drug at all. It's a mineral — part of the same family of minerals that includes sodium and potassium.

I'm talking about *lithium aspartate or lithium orotate* — completely safe minerals you can pick up at any health food store for about 26 cents.

So safe in fact, one healer has used them to treat Alzheimer's for the last 31 years without reporting a single significant side effect. Try to get those kinds of results from prescription drugs!

But even more astounding than the decades-long safety record of these two minerals is how powerful they really are...

Major Alzheimer's Pathways BLOCKED

The FDA-approved Alzheimer's drug Namenda® has been touted as the solution, but in reality, it blocks only ONE Alzheimer pathway.

Meanwhile, *Lithium aspartate* and *orotate* have been shown to block major pathways in recent studies.

Not to mention Namenda® runs about $4.84 a day — almost 20 times what it costs you for your 26-cent-a-day lithium tablets.

But here's the worst part — one of Namenda's® most common side effects is...*confusion!?*

That means this drug that supposedly treats confusion is actually causing it!

Unbelievable, you say. Well, this is coming straight from the normally tight-lipped FDA's own website.

Now, you have to ask yourself: "Why haven't I heard about this before?"

Because of modern medicine's "Golden Rule" — *those with the gold make the rules.* And here's the bottom line...

If they can't patent it, they can't profit...so they don't want it.

Lithium aspartate and lithium orotate are minerals. Which means they cannot be patented. And without a patent Big Pharma cannot profit.

Of course, this is the kind of straightforward answer you'll never get from them. They're too busy counting the money they make from your misery and strong-arming you into paying 20 times more for a drug that is only 1/6th as potent and can actually CAUSE the very thing you are trying to treat.

Isn't it about time you turned the tables in your favor? Discover hundreds of Mother Nature's Real Life Cures...

It doesn't matter if it's Alzheimer's, high cholesterol, hormone replacement therapy, pain reduction or any of hundreds of other concerns there is *always* information on a safe and natural alternative. But discovering them is another matter entirely.

That's why Dr. Wright wants to give you his world-famous 8-VOLUME *Library of Food & Vitamin Cures*...absolutely FREE. He wants to show you how to get healthier than you ever dreamed...*without drugs*.

More on that in a minute, but first I want to tell you how the answer to diabetes may be hiding in your spice rack...keep reading.

CHAPTER TWO

Stop diabetes in its tracks!

It's a solution so simple and effective it's positively <u>revolutionary</u>.

Until recently, type II diabetics thought they had no choice but to overpay for dangerous prescription drugs and endure their dangerous side effects:

- **extreme weakness**
- **muscle pain**
- **trouble breathing**
- **and even heart arrhythmia**

But it doesn't have to be this way.

There's an all-natural, completely underused treatment for type II diabetes. But don't expect to hear about it from your doctor. Not because he's keeping it from you. He simply doesn't know about it. And Big Pharma doesn't want him to know about it. Because, as you know...

If they can't patent it, they can't profit... so they don't want it!

You see, a natural substance can't be patented. And without a patent, Big Pharma can't profit.

Of course, this is the kind of straightforward answer you'll never get from them. They're too busy strong-arming you into paying far too much for synthetic drugs that may actually *harm you*.

So what's this miracle treatment? The cure is so simple it may shock you...

It's an isolated extract of cinnamon...no, not some exotic variety but a *common household cinnamon*.

This cinnamon contains a very powerful nutrient called methylhydroxychalcone polymer — MHCP for short. And new research has shown that MHCP closely mimics human insulin. Better still, it helps your own insulin control blood sugar much more efficiently.

What does this mean to you?

It means many diabetics may be able to <u>say goodbye to drugs forever</u>. For many others, MHCP could completely stop the progression of type II diabetes...*stop it dead in its tracks...*

It's proving a huge help for type I diabetes too

As type I diabetics know too well, injected insulin causes its own set of problems. But proper use of MHCP may reduce the amount you have to use.

So you should just start sprinkling cinnamon on everything you eat, right?

Well, not really. You need to know *exactly* how much to use, how to work it safely into your current program — and how to *remove the toxins* found in natural cinnamon. (No need to worry if you're just flavoring foods with cinnamon, but anyone using more than 1/4 teaspoon daily needs to learn how to "filter" it).

Jonathan Wright, MD, would like to send you all the details about how to use MHCP to whip diabetes in your FREE BONUS *Library of Food & Vitamin Cures* — a life-changing set of 8 reports. You'll learn about hundreds of safe, natural, affordable and effective secrets for a healthier and longer life.

But keep reading to learn about a true

The delicious discovery that slashes stroke risk by 40%

Just about everyone loves it and Dr. Wright has been urging us to eat *more* of it for decades.

Get the facts on a massive 12-year study that reports the same thing Dr. Wright has been saying for years! If Americans ate *just one more serving* per day of this delicious food, it could prevent 40% of all strokes from ever happening! That's because it's rich in a powerful nutrient that strengthens and rejuvenates *every blood vessel in your body*.

You're probably having some tonight. Just eat a little more.

Full details are in the FREE BONUS *Library of Food & Vitamin Cures* Dr. Wright has set aside for you.

cancer cure that might be growing in your vegetable garden right now...

CHAPTER THREE

The astonishing vegetable cure for cancer

Could a true cancer cure with a *100% success rate* get covered up?

Even if it has 80,000 success stories and a 26-year track record?

Sadly, that's exactly what happened. And it might have stayed that way forever if not for Dr. Jonathan Wright's refusal to stay quiet about it.

You see, it turns out than an extract from eggplant can cure — that's *cure*, not just improve — the majority of non-melanoma skin cancers (squamous and basal cell cancers), *usually in three months or less*. This may seem like an outrageous claim, but researchers have known about these incredible results for over 20 years.

It might have remained a secret for another two decades if Dr. Wright hadn't published the research — and dared tell the truth: *It's a cure!*

Just look at the proof straight from Royal London Hospital's double-blind, placebo controlled study…

Using a form of eggplant extract called BEC5, doctors treated both invasive and non-invasive non-melanoma skin cancers. The results were equal to those resulting from invasive surgery, minus the scars.

And doctors concluded: "In our view and experience, BEC5 is…safe and effective…it is a cost-effective treatment for both primary and secondary skin cancer."

EMPHYSEMA strangled Erwin until his face was a dull, mottled blue…

But Dr. Wright simply asked him to inhale a common nutrient, and Erwin was a new man.

"The lung doctor can hardly believe how well I'm doing," says Erwin. "He's going to use [your treatment] for all his other patients."

Even more importantly, follow-up research on patients who used BEC5 shows once their cancer went away, it did not recur.

But that's just the tip of the iceberg. You'll hear how patient records kept since the 1980s show an estimated...

Success in 80,000 cases with ZERO return of the cancer

Over 80,000 patients have used it successfully. Microscopic analysis consistently shows death of all cancer cells. Better yet, no cancer has ever returned.

Best of all, BEC5 does not kill any healthy human cells. With microscopic precision, it selects and *eliminates only the cancer cells*. Healthy cells are not affected in any way by the treatment.

A major breakthrough? *You bet it is*.

More than a million new cases of non-melanoma skin cancer will be diagnosed in the U.S. this year alone.

Yet this same eggplant breakthrough is so safe and effective, it can even be used cosmetically — to eradicate age spots, sun spots and "pre-cancers" called actinic keratoses.

It's non-invasive, non-toxic and so easy to use, you can do it at home. Simple as smoothing on skin cream.

So how did our mighty medical press miss this one?

How come you never saw anything about it...not in magazines...not on TV...not even on the Internet?

Want to sing it with me? *Those with the gold make the rules*! And this astonishingly cheap, effective cancer cure has just one unfortunate drawback...

It threatens the pocketbooks of pharmaceutical firms, dermatology clinics and plastic surgeons. (And the eggplant lobby isn't nearly as powerful as you might imagine.)

But Jonathan Wright, M.D. isn't content to sit by and watch Big Pharma line its coffers while a true natural cure exists. That's why he would like to send you all the details in a brand-new FREE Report — "The Astonishing Eggplant Cure for Cancer." It's just one of 8 FREE Reports he has for you in your free BONUS *Library of Food & Vitamin Cures*...revealing hundreds of equally safe,

Doctors laud
Jonathan Wright, M.D.

"...doing things drug companies never imagined possible..."

"[Dr. Wright] proved that a lone physician, whose cause is true, can prevail... Medical history will judge after this: 'Wright makes might!'...Your scientific accomplishments are no less impressive: You were among the first physicians to embrace orthomolecular [natural] medicine and you write about it with intelligence...Your medical discoveries and applications are numerous... And your... newsletter, *Nutrition & Healing*, has kept the American people abreast of the real progress in this field...Thank you, Dr. Wright."

~ From the text of the Linus Pauling Award, given to Dr. Wright by fellow physicians

"Using the most common nutrients on earth, Dr. Jonathan Wright is doing things that drug companies never imagined possible. Listen to him. It could add years to your life."

~ Randall E. Wilkinson, MD, Coeur d'Alene, ID

"Dr. Wright is one of the smartest clinicians I have ever met. Alternative doctors everywhere know and respect him. His remarkable insights and medical wisdom have proven miraculous for so many."

~ Michael Berger, N.D.

ANGINA PAIN held John in its grip for three agonizing years...

His wife was understandably terrified. *"[John's] father died of a heart attack at age 55,"* she told him. *"John is 53!"* But within just two weeks, John reduced his angina...and after six months he was off all medications and totally free of chest pain. Now he can run two miles without a twinge! Let Dr. Wright show you what did it.

natural, affordable and effective secrets for a healthier and longer life.

Keep reading to learn about the sugar cane shocker that is shaking the medical world...

CHAPTER FOUR

Spectacular sugar cane cures outdo cholesterol drugs

They've told you that *all sugar* is bad, but surprise...Dr. Wright has discovered that, much like fats, there are "bad" and "good" sugars, and the difference can transform your health in days — *or even minutes.*

Bad sugars attract dangerous germs. You see, sugar isn't just sweet for us — germs love it too. The sugar in your body sends out chemical signals that draw them like moths to a flame. By reading the "sugar code" on your cell walls, these pathogens target cells all over your body. But what if you could turn that secret code *against* your microbial enemies? Thanks to Dr. Wright, now you can, with...

'GOOD' sugars that disable germs

These "exotic" varieties aren't found in table sugar, but they do show up in small quantities in certain fruits, like cranberries.

Their molecules are just a little different, but it makes a *huge* difference to germs...

Instead of just waiting to be eaten, these *good* sugars overwhelm germs by jamming their chemical "radar" and blocking the cellular receptors these pathogens grab hold of (kind of like coating your cells with Teflon). Suddenly, germs have a hard time even finding your cells — but if they do manage to locate a few, they're too slippery to cling to.

Because they can't hang on, your body fluids then wash these germs away harmlessly. It's not too good to be true...Dr. Wright has found sugars that do exactly this.

Take "Sugar X" for example. It looks and tastes a lot like ordinary table sugar, but actually *disables* bacteria...

Conquer tooth decay *with sugar?* Strange but true

To start with, researchers created a gum made from Sugar X. Amazingly, people who chewed it got *80% less tooth decay*, even though they didn't change their eating habits. But it gets better...

In addition to washing out germs, it

apparently works the same magic on *pollutants, pollen grains* and other allergens that attach to your mucous membranes, triggering hay fever and asthma attacks. Suddenly, all those micro-particles get 'unstuck' and slip away.

Now maybe you're asking, can the same thing work for more serious diseases? That's a big "yes."

For example, a colleague of Dr. Wright's placed Sugar X in a nose spray and gave it to people with chronic ear and sinus infections. He reported lifelong sufferers were shocked to find...

Sinus and ear infections
SLASHED BY 93%

Yes, this same sugar 'unsticks' the germs in your nose, sinuses and ear canals! Spray it in, wait a bit, blow your nose, and away go the bacteria.

You better believe I've tried it myself. You can feel the difference *in minutes*. If you're a sinus sufferer, or know a child tortured by ear infections, think of what this means. Instead of being doomed to a lifetime of antibiotics and all the nasty side-effects they bring...no more diarrhea and cramps, no more yeast overgrowths, no more fatigue, *no more suffering, period.*

But that's just the start, because Sugar X has proven equally miraculous for asthma and hay fever sufferers.

In addition to washing out germs, it apparently works the same magic on *pollutants, pollen grains* and other allergens that attach to your mucous membranes, triggering hay fever and asthma attacks. Suddenly, all those micro-particles get 'unstuck' and slip away.

And there's similar sweet news about BLADDER AND URINARY INFECTIONS

If you or your spouse has ever suffered these painful attacks, I don't have to tell you what antibiotics *can't* do. They *can't* keep the infection from bouncing back as soon the drugs stop.

Worse, the germs quickly gain *immunity* to the antibiotic. Drugs like penicillin that *used* to work well must now be taken at *triple* the old dosage. In a frightening number of new cases, they can't kill the bugs at all...

'Sugar M' washes out bugs that resist the most powerful antibiotics

The scientific name for this miraculous sugar is *D-Mannose*. And it has already proved a godsend for *hundreds* of patients at Dr. Wright's clinic, and readers of Dr. Wright's exclusive *Nutrition & Healing* newsletter who have tried it themselves. In most cases, patients are infection free in less than 48 hours. The bacteria become so slippery they can no longer cling to your cell walls. *You literally flush them down the toilet.*

More good news. These healing sugars even taste delicious, yet...

They don't make you fat, because they 'slip-slide' right through your digestive system. They can even help you *lose weight...*

Are you starting to see why so many doctors are starting to study Dr. Wright's theories? *His solutions don't just stave off disease, they wipe it out for good.*

Yet all this is just the beginning. Think even bigger. Like *heart disease...*

Cut cholesterol with SUGAR CANE?!

Actually, it's even more astonishing than

that...

Even if you've been blissfully ignoring your doctor's advice for years, drinking, eating the wrong foods, not getting enough exercise...

Maybe you won't have to pay the piper after all. To a stunned world, Dr. Wright recently revealed details about an all-natural sugar cane extract that's now doing patients more benefit than the latest cholesterol-controlling statin drugs.

Unlike dangerous drugs that simply lower cholesterol, this harmless extract does just about everything your heart could desire. Several studies show that it can:

✔ **Cut TOTAL cholesterol as much as 17%...**

✔ **Slash LDL cholesterol by 25%...**

✔ **Raise HDL ('good') cholesterol up to 29%...**

✔ **Drop dangerous triglycerides as much as 18%...**

Getting the picture? Your *whole circulatory system* just got a second chance...

No drug known to science can match this

Skeptical? So were a lot of scientists. They proceeded to test the sugar cane extract against top prescription drugs — substances with some very dangerous side-effects. In three different double-blind, placebo-controlled studies, they put it up against

Reduce systolic blood pressure by 20, 30...EVEN 40 POINTS

Fred K. wasn't even 50 years old, but when he came to Dr. Wright, his blood pressure was 170 over 110. He was taking a calcium channel-blocker and a beta-blocker — and the drugs seemed to be his only hope.

I'd already cut out all the added salt," says his wife Susan. "I eliminated the high-salt foods, and switched us to decaffeinated coffee. We cut out all the alcohol, too, except a little beer and wine. But his blood pressure just kept going up!"

But Fred soon dropped his blood pressure to normal, tossed out both drugs, and Dr. Wright will show you how to do the same, in your FREE BONUS *Library of Food & Vitamin Cures.*

prevastatin (Prevachol®), lovastatin (Mevacor®), simvastatin (Zocor®)...

The sugar cane miracle whomped them all. More benefits, no side-effects, and all at a slender fraction of the cost. The results leave little room for doubt.

Yet it's so safe, even diabetics use it with no harmful side effects

In fact, it's been carefully tested on people with type II diabetes and has proved totally safe, with *no* adverse impact on glucose control.

Yes, even though it's a sugar cane extract. Because this remarkable substance has practically *zero* carbohydrate content. (Technically, it's not even a sugar.) And this most amazing of "sugar cures" has even more tricks up its sleeve...

For example, it reduces blood clot risk *without* aspirin...

Meaning you get the lifesaving benefit *without* the risk of intestinal bleeding and osteoporosis that aspirin therapy carries. But there's even more it can do for you, as you'll learn in your FREE BONUS *Library of Food & Vitamin Cures.* (You'll also learn exactly how to find Sugar X and Sugar M.) And in case you're wondering…

Why didn't my own doctor tell me about this?

Great question. I know this much…it's not your doctor's fault. Incredibly, nutritional cures and natural medicine are hardly even mentioned in medical school. And doctors are often just pawns in the big-money game of corporate medicine.

That's exactly why many thousands of caring physicians — alternative and traditional-minded doctors alike — are flocking to Dr. Wright's seminars and subscribing to *Nutrition & Healing.*

Because he's *always* pushing beyond medicine's old "comfort zone." Challenging smug assumptions. Coming up with dazzling new solutions to puzzles that have eluded tradition-bound doctors for years.

This is also where many doctors found out for the first time about how standard prostate therapy is *encouraging* cancer and…

TURNING MEN INTO WOMEN. Did that get your attention? Turn to Chapter Five…

Ultimate prostate treatment shrinks swelling, may prevent cancer, protects manhood

Prostate drugs can flatten your sex life, but at least they're good for your prostate...right?

Are you sitting down? Researchers at the University of Southern California recently tested this assumption, and the results couldn't have been more alarming.

As recorded in the *British Journal of Cancer*, they studied 52 men with high PSA scores. First they gave the men baseline biopsies to make sure there were no signs of cancer.

Then they gave 27 of the men a one-year course of finasteride (Proscar®), the standard drug for benign prostate problems. The other 25 were given nothing.

When the year was up, researchers gave each man a second biopsy. Guess what they found?

Nearly 30% of the men taking Proscar® developed prostate tumors

Yet tumors were found in only one of the 25 men taking nothing. Which raises the obvious question...

How can this be? How could our "best" prostate drugs turn out to be cancer fertilizer?

The reason is more alarming still...

As Dr. Wright told his readers years ago, these drugs are literally turning men into women.

You see, Proscar® works by blocking the normal 'pathway' of your testosterone. Ordinarily, some of your testosterone turns into a slightly different hormone, called DHT (dihydrotestosterone)...and swollen prostates often contain high levels of DHT. So drug firms assumed DHT was causing the trouble.

They developed powerful drugs like Proscar® to suppress DHT production. Sound

Months of infection gone in 2 days

Dear Dr. Wright:

"My wife recently had a urinary infection. I had just read your article on [Sugar M] and quickly ordered some. Although the physician estimated my wife had the infection for many months, it took only a couple of days [on this new treatment] and she felt better."

— *T. S. M.*

like a good idea? Maybe, until you consider what else happens when you block this process. When your body can't make DHT...

Lots of testosterone turns into estrogen

Yes, estrogen...the female hormone! Now, scientists have known for decades that the human body creates estrogen out of testosterone. (That's how women's bodies make it.) And a little estrogen is normal in men. But when a man's estrogen ratio gets too high...

The entire male edifice crumbles

Your erections wilt, your libido sinks, you can develop a form of diabetes, your heart risk rockets...

Is it really any wonder you're more likely to get cancer too?

Yet drug firms continue to make billions selling these stealth sex change pills. Even though Dr. Wright has pioneered a much more powerful way to *turn off* your prostate swelling and *turn on* your cancer-fighting genes.

You'll find Dr. Wright's famous program for ending benign prostate swelling in your FREE BONUS *Library of Food & Vitamin*

Congestive heart failure weighed upon Helen like a giant rock...

She was bedridden and her lungs were so full of fluid, she couldn't even sleep without being propped up. But Dr. Wright soon had her sleeping like a baby and feeling so strong, *she even started gardening again!* What did he know that others didn't?

Get full details about the nutrient treatment that saved her life in your FREE BONUS *Library of Food & Vitamin Cures*!

Cures. It's breathtakingly simple. As you'll see...

You may be wasting your money on saw palmetto

Sure, it can bring some relief, but it doesn't correct the cause of the problem. No man on earth ever suffered from a saw palmetto deficiency. But plenty of men are short on a couple of common nutrients. They cost peanuts, yet they're all you may need to shrink swollen tissue and to urinate like a teenager.

Then, Dr. Wright will show how adding just one more cheap mineral to this incredibly simple program can virtually armor-plate your prostate against cancer.

Is prostate cancer a nutritional disease?

Some so-called experts scoffed when Dr. Wright suggested this. Just as scurvy is caused by a vitamin C deficiency, Dr. Wright wondered if prostate cancer might be triggered by a selenium deficiency.

Too easy to be true? But just months ago, researchers at Indiana University provided stunning confirmation. They showed that selenium activates and protects a gene called p53. And this gene instructs your cells to repair damaged DNA. If a deficiency knocks this gene out of action, cancer becomes far more likely.

This selenium discovery is so powerful it could also be a key to preventing lung, breast and colon cancer too, all for just pennies a day. Are you starting to see how simple and safe the world's most powerful cures can be? And thanks to Dr. Wright, now it's equally easy to defeat any kind of pain...

Every man who feels even a little 'behind the curve' should know the *truth* about testosterone. So RSVP today to get your **FREE BONUS** *Library of Food & Vitamin Cures.*

We're not even close to done here. Next, learn about how Dr. Wright is blowing the doors off a shocking medical cover up...

CHAPTER SIX

What drug firms call 'hormone replacement therapy' is really HORSE URINE therapy

I t's true. The chemical content is so
dangerous, it's a miracle millions more
women didn't get breast cancer. Yet for
nearly 20 years, Dr. Wright has been
prescribing a safe and truly miraculous
answer. So why haven't you heard about it
until now?

It's time to end the coverup. Despite what
drug firms would have you believe, today's
HRT crisis is not a surprise. The inherent
dangers revealed in recent clinical trials were
suspected for decades...

And Dr. Wright first sounded the warning
20 YEARS AGO.

That's right...Nearly two decades ago,

Dr. Wright told his patients and readers why conventional 'Hormone Replacement Therapy' was a recipe for disaster. And he pioneered the only sane solution.

Millions of women might have been spared needless suffering...

And many lives might have been saved — if drug firms hadn't drowned out Dr. Wright's message in a sea of advertising. Here's what they conveniently left out of all those celebrity TV commercials:

■ **HUSH UP #1:** The HRT advertised on TV and used by researchers in the recent

Dr. Wright tells us about an herb that "repairs" pancreas cells so they make their own insulin!

In your FREE BONUS *Library of Food & Vitamin Cures*, you'll also learn full details about this herbal discovery that's helping type I and type II diabetics combat this deadly disease. In controlled studies on diabetics, this natural discovery cut their insulin needs by 50%. More amazing still, lab tests on diabetic subjects show it can even...

Women's Health Initiative study does not replace human hormones with anything resembling human hormones.

■ **HUSH UP #2:** Standard HRT uses molecules never before found in human bodies. In fact, the best-selling 'HRT' contains horse hormones extracted from horse urine.

■ **HUSH UP #3:** When you flood your body with molecular gunk that nature never intended to be there, damage is virtually guaranteed. You may as well pour molasses into your car's gas tank.

Reverse diabetes damage in as little as 20 days

Time and again, the pancreas actually regained the ability to make insulin. The number of insulin-producing cells in the pancreas increased, meaning the damage was being repaired! More research is needed, but this could prove to be the biggest diabetes breakthrough of our time. The herb is readily available, cheap and carries no harmful side-effects.

At this point, some patients ask "But aren't horse hormones natural?" Sure they are, and they're fine for mares. But do you wear a saddle?

Let's look at what's actually in this stuff:

Prempro®, the substance tested by the Women's Health Initiative, consists of two different drugs — Premarin® and Provera®. The main ingredient in Premarin…yep, that's short for "pregnant mares"…is a horse hormone called equilin. Nature never put a speck of equilin in any human woman, and for excellent reason.

Its effects on your uterine lining are 1,000 times stronger than human estrogen. No wonder it increases your cancer risk!

Yet it's the best-selling drug of our time.

The second component in Prempro is called Provera and it's not progesterone. It's an artificial molecule patented in the 1940s and it's not even natural to horses. (No wonder it's proven hazardous to your heart.)

But the problem isn't just Prempro.

More than 25 other so-called "HRT" products have been approved by the FDA.

Some call themselves 'natural,' but even these do not replicate the estrogen of a healthy woman. Here's why...Human estrogen is actually a blend of many different molecules.

Chief among these are estriol, estrone and estradiol. (Tough to pronounce, but remember them — these three little words could save your life!) And they've got to be properly balanced or you're inviting big trouble.

It's turn out, women with breast cancer tend to be low on estriol and high on estradiol.

Yet many patented 'HRT' products are HIGH in estradiol. Want to guess what they're likely to do?

But Dr. Wright's 'alternative' is THE REAL THING

It's called BIO-IDENTICAL HORMONE THERAPY. And it's not an "alternative" at all — because it replicates the exact same estrogen balance that's been keeping women healthy for 200,000 years.

Dr. Wright has been using it for 20 years, prescribing it for thousands of women. The incredible relief they have reported is a matter of public record. In many cases, these women have replaced lost bone mass, come back from life-threatening heart conditions — and in all this time, only a few of all these thousands of women have ever been diagnosed with cancer. (That's far lower than the national average of one in eight women.)

After all is said and done, isn't the safest, sanest treatment always the one that's friendliest to your body?

So why aren't YOU getting Dr. Wright's therapy?

You easily could. It's available throughout America, and his FREE BONUS *Library of Food & Vitamin Cures* will direct you to a doctor who can prescribe it. But your doctor may not have heard about it...

Because that's the way our drug-centered health system works. Mainstream doctors prescribe what drug companies promote. Drug companies won't promote what they can't patent — and your body chemistry can't be patented. And that's not even the worst of it...

The FDA — the government department you'd like to believe has your best interests at heart — is actually working in cahoots with

Big Pharma. (After all, drug money keeps the FDA in business.) In fact, just recently the FDA caved to pressure from one pharmaceutical giant to try to block the compounding of hormone treatments that contain estriol.

That's right…our own FDA is trying to block access to vital treatment options. Of course, Dr. Wright is fighting to get Congress to step in against this outrage… but it's tough to win against Big Pharma's billions.

With our own government and giant corporations conspiring to keep natural cures from you, it's easy to understand why Dr. Wright's breakthroughs, like his incredible natural cure for joint pain (Chapter Seven)…the one with an almost perfect success rate…remain a well-kept secret…

The secret culprit behind your joint pain

"I know there aren't any cures," Theresa C. told Dr. Wright. "I don't expect some of my joints will ever look normal again."

But Theresa was wrong and is she ever happy for that. Before long, her pain *and* her joint deformities were almost entirely gone. She stopped her 12 daily pain pills because she just didn't need them.

Astonishing? But to Dr. Wright, this "miracle" was quite routine. For years, he's seen the same treatment for inflammatory arthritis heal patient after patient...

His success rate is close to perfect

That's almost unheard-of in medicine — and new research now confirms Dr. Wright is onto yet another huge breakthrough. He's recognized the healing potential in a little known discovery by Dr. James Breneman — the secret culprit hiding behind a large percentage of joint pain *and more than 50% of all undiagnosed illness...*

It's called low-level food sensitivity. And what it means is that your body can't tolerate certain foods. Oh, you won't break out in hives, but they *will* trigger immune reactions. Before long, you might come down with a full blown autoimmune condition, like arthritis, lupus, asthma, colitis, Graves' disease, chronic fatigue...

Yet if you simply stop the offending food, the problem melts away like snow in the spring. *Want proof?* Dr. Wright's track record is quite convincing by itself, but now there's plenty more evidence too...

100 patients totally cured of "incurable" lupus

You'll hear about an Australian colleague of Dr. Wright's — Dr. Christopher Reading of Sydney — who treated 100 people with so-called "incurable" lupus. All of them had full-blown symptoms (which include joint pain, fever and skin rash) and they weren't just

Cut health costs in half ...and your suffering down to *nothing*

Can you really cut your healthcare costs in half? Before you dismiss this as hype, let's look at the facts. A few years ago, a major corporate study on a large group of people proved that...

Just one breakthrough used by Dr. Wright cut all their long-term health problems *by more than 50%*...

Just one! That's how incredibly powerful Dr. Wright's "new medicine" is.

That's why he's such a legend among so many doctors *and* patients.

And that's why I urge you to seize upon his *new* approach to healing today...

Stop treating your pain only to see it come bouncing back...

Start eliminating the cause and feel your entire body bounce back, often faster than you ever dared imagine!

It all starts as soon as you claim your FREE BONUS *Library of Food & Vitamin Cures*...

And if just one of his discoveries can slice your health problems in half, imagine what they *all* could do for you. I've only had space in this book to scratch the surface of what you'll find in your FREE BONUS Library.

You'll get full details — and Dr. Wright's comprehensive instructions — covering everything you'll read on these pages and so much more, like:

- **SHRINKING UTERINE FIBROIDS.** This ancient Chinese herbal therapy could make more than *half* of all fibroid surgeries unnecessary.

- **ASTONISHING ASTHMA FACT.** Dr. Wright has found great success with asthmatic kids through the use of ONE vitamin. Let him show you how.

- **VARICOSE VEIN VANISHING ACT.** Don't just suffer and blame your heredity. You're probably just not getting enough of a very important food! The remedy is *so* easy.

- **THE BURSITIS BUSTER.** Often bursitis is simply a signal that you're *deficient in good old vitamin B12*. Supplement correctly and all the aching can go away.

- **THE PSORIASIS SENSATION.** If you're suffering, you've got to try Dr. Wright's solution.

All these life-giving discoveries and hundreds more, FREE

To claim all 8 lifesaving volumes of FREE BONUS *Library of Food & Vitamin Cures,* just fill out your GIFT CERTIFICATE and mail it in the enclosed postage-free envelope.

imagining it. *They all tested positive for lupus in blood tests.*

Yet reports show their symptoms soon vanished and *five years later all blood tests came up negative.* They were cured. And all they really did was take some vitamins and cut a few foods from their diet...

Eliminating all grains except rice and corn. You see, these lupus sufferers all shared a sensitivity to *gluten* and *gliadin,* proteins contained in wheat, rye, barley, spelt and oats, but *not* in corn or rice. And now, a brand-new study reveals it's...

The secret tormentor of 90 million Americans

Decades after Dr. Wright first championed the cause, a brand-new, landmark book just published this year links this same grain sensitivity to joint pain, cancer, depression, brain disorders...even osteoporosis. The study estimates that as many as 90 million Americans are suffering without even suspecting the cause...

And genetic research clinches it. Cutting-edge research reveals that many people with autoimmune diseases share certain genetic commonalities that are *known markers for extreme gluten intolerance.*

And Dr. Wright has found that *when he treats the food intolerance,* the other problems fade away...without any need for prednisone or other immune-system destroying medicines. *The results are fantastic.*

Is YOUR PAIN from grain?

You may be secretly sensitive to grain, or dairy or something else you never suspected — but why guess? Get full details on how to test yourself for food sensitivity *and* clear up the problem for good in your FREE BONUS *Library of Food & Vitamin Cures,* where you'll also discover how to protect yourself from the number-one cause of vision loss (keep reading)...

CHAPTER EIGHT

Could the secret to saving your eyesight be found in a bowl of chili?

If you're trying to fight vision loss, you don't need a prescription — and, please stay out of the operating room! Because you'll find more effective ways to save your vision in your kitchen than you would in any hospital or pharmacy.

It's true…there are simple, safe natural ways to fight the number one cause of vision loss — age-related macular degeneration or ARMD.

But there's no time to waste. Even the Director of National Eye Institute recently stated that age-related macular degeneration (ARMD) will soon become an epidemic.

You read right…he said *epidemic*. A word used to describe AIDS, type II diabetes, and

See clearly

Since 1985, Dr. Wright's breakthrough nutritional treatment has reliably saved 70% of all patients with apparently "incurable" dry macular degeneration by stopping the progression of the disease or in many cases actually reversing much of the vision loss. Here's what patients and doctors are saying about it...

"After a month...no trace of macular degeneration"

"I consulted with two doctors at Eye Associates, and then two specialists at the Virginia Mason Clinic. They told me I had macular degeneration and there wasn't anything that could be done...it would just be getting worse. Within a month of starting [Dr. Wright's treatment], my eyes returned to normal. When I went back to my eye doctor...he stated there was no trace left of macular degeneration."

—*Joan P.*

"As an added bonus my hearing improved"

"Television was easier to see and reading became easier. I had to go back to using the

in 30 days

glasses that I had gotten a year earlier as they were not as strong. As an added bonus, I noticed that my hearing had improved some... I had to turn the TV volume down several notches."

—*Gertrude G.*

"Dr. Wright's secret saved the eyesight of my patients"

"Mostly they were told...that nothing can be done...the prognosis is hopeless. I can testify from clinical experience I have that about seven out of ten of the patients who have come in with this diagnosis...benefitted substantially...what a boon it is to save one's vision!"

—*Dr. Tom Dorman*

Now it's your turn. If you know anyone with this heartbreaking condition or any other age-related degenerative problems, don't wait another day for things to get worse: Do something now while there's time...

Get full details in your FREE BONUS *Library of Food & Vitamin Cures*. RSVP now!

heart disease. This is getting very serious. But now, thanks to Dr. Jonathan Wright, there's hope.

The 'Mineral and Vitamin' ARMD-prevention program that starts in your kitchen

Possibly just the contents in your kitchen (with no digestive aids or IV nutrients) can actually PREVENT the problem, and once it starts....

It begins with simple remedies like homemade chili. That's because high quality red meat, beans, garlic and onions are some of the richest "eye foods" you can eat.

See, with just the right additions to your diet and Dr. Wright's reliable team of eye-saving nutrients, you'll be well on your way to keeping your vision sharp as an eagle.

So no matter what you've heard about macular degeneration, the simple truth is there is a solution, and *you never need to go blind*.

Not a chili fan? Not a problem! As long as you know which vital nutrients (because vitamins and amino acids are involved, too) are missing from your diet, you can easily uncover a whole world of vision-saving recipes. Incredible as it sounds, it's really happening — because Dr. Wright is constantly pushing the envelope. Now, you too will learn to:

✔ **Safeguard your vision** with one delicious food that's the strongest source of eyesight power (but be careful...it's also a popular aphrodisiac)...

Joint pain and depression made George a shell of his former self...

But Dr. Wright detected the shockingly simple cause behind *both*. "George's sense of humor is back, he's smiling and the kids and grandkids are amazed," reports his wife. "*His knees don't hurt any more either*, and he's almost as fun and funny as when we were first married, even though his jokes aren't any better!"

Learn what Dr. Wright did in your FREE BONUS *Library of Food & Vitamin Cures*.

✔ Avoid these 3 prescription vision killers.
3 popular prescription drugs may actually help macular degeneration take over your eyes!? Check this information before filling out your next Rx

✔ Unlock your body's secret ARMD fighter —
in fact, the best way to save your vision is already inside you waiting to work wonders, you just need to know how to use it...

And now, Dr. Wright has compiled his most important research for you in his *Library of Food & Vitamin Cures*. Dr. Wright's famed "food and vitamin remedies" have been showing unparalleled results for decades.

In fact, Dr. Wright's success with ARMD (and many other illnesses) is the reason there's *a six month wait to see him*. And he accomplishes it all for you without prescription pills, invasive surgical procedures, or any of modern medicine's costly side-effects (costly both to your wallet and health)!

Isn't it time you learned about them too right now?

Just sign up today and Dr. Wright will be

pleased to send you 8 FREE BONUS GIFTS detailing all of his most valuable new breakthroughs.

Whether you want to restore your own health, or help a parent, spouse or loved one...this FREE 8-VOLUME BONUS *Library of Food & Vitamin Cures* will show you how to get healthier than you ever dreamed, without surgery, drugs, radiation or anything else more dangerous than natural minerals and nutrients.

CHAPTER NINE

Are your new painkillers *causing* your back pain?

It's really happening. You go to your doctor for back pain and he prescribes the widely hyped new and powerful pain-killers. But despite all those merry commercials singing 'Celebrate! Celebrate!' your pain actually increases...

Are you just imagining it? Nope. This nifty little side effect has been documented by the drug firms themselves. In a significant number of cases, Cox-2 inhibitors have been linked to back pain.

So what good are they? Maybe they're safer than previous painkillers, right?

That was the promise. The reason for their development was to find something safer than aspirin, ibuprofen or acetaminophen. But now, even the ultra-conservative *Journal of the American Medical Association* warns that new studies "raise a cautionary flag about the risk of cardiovascular events."

In plain English:
Watch out for heart attacks.

One of these studies involved 23,408 people. Heart attack rates for those taking the drugs Vioxx® and Celebrex® were so much higher, it couldn't be a coincidence. Initially, the US Food and Drug Administration (FDA) asked the maker of Vioxx to caution doctors...and then the drug's maker removed it from the market altogether...

But who's telling the PATIENTS?
Dr. Wright, that's who

In the pages of his newsletter *Nutrition & Healing*, he was among the first to warn about these dangers. This is also where he broke the shocking news that even when they don't kill, these new drugs work no better than the humblest, cheapest painkiller in human history...

After 100 years of trying, drug makers still can't beat tree bark

Maybe you knew that willow bark was the inspiration for aspirin, the granddaddy of synthetic analgesics. Aspirin doesn't work any better — Bayer developed aspirin simply so they could patent it. But Dr. Wright really rocked the boat when he published clinical data suggesting that even 'fancy' prescription drugs can't beat tree bark!

Check out the details in your FREE BONUS *Library of Food & Vitamin Cures.*

Then discover Dr. Wright's revolutionary program for real SUCCESS WITH ARTHRITIS

Rest assured, Dr. Wright's program

What's hurting you?

■ **Osteoarthritis?** Harry's joints were so swollen, he needed a cane to get out of his chair. But thanks to Dr. Wright, 10 years of pain and swelling soon *vanished.*

■ **Rheumatoid Arthritis?** Theresa was taking 12 pills a day and her joints were so deformed she doubted she'd ever look "normal" again. But before long, both her pain and her deformities were almost entirely gone — and so were the drugs! Dr. Wright's success rate with this treatment is nearly *100%.*

consists of nothing more than taking a few nutrients and changing some eating habits. Yet it results in the most dramatic relief in the history of this stubborn condition. Plus, your FREE BONUS Library will show you...

How 6 years of chronic pain can VANISH IN 30 SECONDS

Susan had been suffering unrelenting, disabling pain, day and night for 6 long years. Until she went to Dr. Wright's Tahoma Clinic. Here, she received a nutritional

- **Migraine?** Joan's faded in just 3 minutes, thanks to Dr. Wright's revolutionary vitamin and mineral treatment. "I still can't believe it," she says. "Three minutes...I felt warm and the pain started to fade." (Better still, thanks to his breakthrough program, they never came back.")

- **Gall Bladder Pain?** Laura's was gone in three days! Let Dr. Wright show you how he eliminates it forever without surgery, in 99% of cases.

    Get these secrets and more in your FREE BONUS *Library of Food & Vitamin Cures* today.

'cocktail,' consisting of nothing more than common vitamins and minerals. And within half a minute, her pain was only a memory! Totally relieved and happy...

She got up from the treatment table and ran across the room!

Amazingly, this kind of relief is more or less typical. You'll learn the formula in your FREE BONUS *Library of Food & Vitamin Cures*. Keep reading to find out why the FDA *banned* the greatest natural cholesterol-buster ever discovered...

CHAPTER TEN

BANNED! Why the FDA *slammed* the door on the greatest natural cholesterol-buster you can get...

It's true. While many Americans are popping risky and expensive statin drugs, the FDA fought to block the sale of a perfectly safe, *natural* source of powerful cholesterol-lowering *lovastatin* ...

It's the same old song and dance... Because the FDA has convinced mainstream medicine that costly drugs are the only answer to all our health worries — despite their dubious track records and often-deadly side effects. This, while muzzling (and muscling) the safe, natural, affordable alternatives.

The drug giants knew they'd be in trouble if word got out about the natural "statin" in one company's red yeast rice product...

Not only did studies show that this specific formulation of this ancient Asian edible slashed cholesterol an average of 40 points in just 3 months, it did so without any side effects whatsoever.

So what did those fat-cat drug executives do? They went to court — then called the FDA...

Their "grounds" for suing? The targeted company's red yeast rice extract contained a natural form of lovastatin, the same active ingredient found in patented Mevacor, one of the major cholesterol drugs...

The first time the drug companies took the red yeast rice maker to court, however, the judge quite rightly threw the case out. But after appealing the case on the grounds that the FDA hadn't officially ratified their natural competition's cholesterol-control claims, they got their verdict...

And with one stroke of the gavel, the company offering a safe, natural, un-patentable solution for managing cholesterol suddenly found itself in violation of Federal law simply for claiming the truth: That its red yeast rice product lowered cholesterol by using the exact same substance prescription drug makers have patented and marked-up a thousand percent or more...

When the decision was handed down, the FDA quickly banned the best known, most proven source of cholesterol-lowering red yeast rice extract — before its makers could regroup and file an appeal or suit of their own. Of course, red yeast rice itself can still be bought from many sources (and it's still a good idea for cholesterol control).

But...unless you'd anticipated the ban and bought a lifetime supply of the one red yeast rice extract proven in federal court to safely slash LDL levels with the same active ingredient in statin drugs, you could very likely end up enduring the risks, expense and side effects of statin drugs for cholesterol control. Which begs the question...

How different would today's medicine be if natural cures were widely known, promoted, and available to all?

From a scientific standpoint, we've only been using patented medications to treat illness and disease for a relatively short time. Yet humankind has practiced medicine for

I realize this is a mind-bender, but do your loved ones a favor...

If they seem to be losing their mental *or* visual sharpness, don't write it off to Father Time. Check out the proof in your FREE BONUS *Library of Food & Vitamin Cures*. And find out why Dr. Wright is such a legend among patients who thought they were just feeling their age. Like...

When Susan's husband started leaving his socks in the fridge...

...she was merely worried. But then he came back from a fishing trip minus the fish, his boat and his dog, *they both* decided to see Dr. Wright.

Vincent thought he was "losing it," but it turned out he was actually missing *the stomach acid* he needed to break down his food. And without it, h*is brain cells* weren't being "fed" the nutrients they depend on. He's sharp as a razor now!

Full details are waiting in your FREE BONUS Library. Respond today.

thousands of years in every corner of the globe. Is it so unbelievable to think that during that vast stretch of time, no one ever learned anything of value about how to prevent, treat, and cure disease?

Of course it isn't. In fact, yesterday's doctors were on the right track — they knew that the cure for every imaginable disease must exist someplace in the natural world...

The truth is, countless numbers of the world's greatest healers were discovered and used ages before there was ever such thing as a patent — or an FDA. These cures are just as effective in this day and age — and would be curing people by the millions if there'd been as much study, promotion and exposure behind them as there have been for risky prescription drugs.

Thankfully, you no longer need to be held "hostage" by big money Corporate Medicine

Your FREE 8-Volume *Library of Food & Vitamin Cures* will show you Dr. Wright's proven secrets for getting healthier than ever...without costly and dangerous drugs. It's waiting just for you...RSVP today.

But first, you must read Chapter Eleven
before you eat another veggie burger…

The Soy Myth — Read this before you eat one more veggie burger

Nowadays you'll have no problem finding soy products at your local grocery store. Soy milk, soy cheese, soy meat balls, soy infant formula, even soy ice cream line the shelves. And, while 10 short years ago it would hardly have seemed possible, today soy products have nearly achieved mainstream acceptance.

And it's healthy, right?

Actually, the answer is more complicated than you think. And the truth? It might just shock you.

Did you know...

An infant fed soy formula is getting the *hormonal equivalent of a birth control pill per day.*

Until the 1930s, the only place in the USA where you could find soybeans was at your local hardware store — in your paint and varnish.

Even after rigorous chemical processing, soy contains substances that can possibly cause *breast cancer, serious nutritional deficiencies, and even accelerated brain aging!*

Two of the FDA's own experts warn that the safety concerns regarding soy are still

Start feeling the difference in months, days...*or minutes*

CHRONIC FATIGUE FALLS AWAY.

"My old energy's back, I've been chomping at the bit to do everything I've not been able to do!"

— *Kathy C.*

ANXIETY VANISHES.

"It's unbelievably less. I feel better all over, as well as being less anxious."

—*Victor H.*

AGING BODIES SURGE WITH NEW ENERGY.

"I not only have more energy, but I've

'largely unanswered.'

Is soy protein a kind of Dr. Jekyll and Mr. Hyde?

Here's the truth. *There are some undeniable benefits to eating soy.* It's high in protein. Low in saturated fat. It's easy on the stomach for some folks — especially babies. And, it works as a meat and dairy substitute.

But like Dr. Jekyll's flip personality, soy has a dark and possibly dangerous side that

noticed that most of my joint aches are gone. I'm seeing a little more clearly and I'll swear my memory is a little better."

— *Grace L.*

HYPERACTIVE KIDS BECOME "NORMAL & BRIGHT."

School authorities wanted to put little Jeremy B. on Ritalin. (No wonder. It turned out the school received about $1,000 in federal funds for each kid they put on the drug!) But Jeremy's treatment required no drugs at all. Later his teacher said, "*[he's] not hyperactive at all, just normal and bright.*" Find out what he did in your FREE Bonus reports…

few people know about.

To start, unlike other legumes, soybeans aren't safe to eat when picked fresh. They're actually toxic. And in laboratory tests in animals, soybeans have been shown to cause everything from cancer to birth defects.

In order to remove the harmful toxins mentioned above, manufacturers must use harsh chemical processing. The beans are subject to acid baths and extreme heat, then they're spray dried to produce a high-protein powder. Next, to improve the taste of the soy powder, artificial flavorings such as MSG, preservatives, sweeteners, emulsifiers, and synthetic nutrients are added.

But manufacturers don't stop there...

Carcinogens called nitrites are also added to soy products during the spray drying process. These harmful chemicals are found in hot dogs and other fast foods...and they've been known since the dark ages to cause cancer. Plus, after all that...

Despite nearly $500,000,000.00 dollars in funding, nobody's figured out how to remove all the toxins from soybeans

That's right. There's not enough money

in the world that can make soybeans completely safe to eat.

The problem is, manufacturers can't get rid of all of the soybean's natural toxins. One especially dangerous toxin, called a trypsin inhibitor, can interfere with digestion and could theoretically cause cancer in humans. And, it's been proven to slow the growth of rats in laboratory tests.

The big question still looming for experts is...*does it inhibit growth in children?*

Scientists can't say for sure yet. But it makes you worry doesn't it? And I imagine you want 'both sides' of the soy story — all the available hard facts — *before pouring that soy milk onto your kids' or grandkids' cereal!*

Post-menopausal women who eat soy may be at greater risk for osteoporosis

Processed soy powder also contains residual phytic acid; a substance experts know *blocks the absorption of calcium, magnesium, zinc, and other essential minerals in the intestinal tract.*

In feeding experiments, a soy-based diet requires supplementation with vitamins E, K, D, B12, and creates significant

DEFICIENCIES in copper, iron, zinc, magnesium, and calcium. This revelation is especially important for post-menopausal women. By eating quantities of soy, you could be putting yourself at risk for serious nutritional deficiencies and osteoporosis. But that's not the only concern for women eating soy...

Researchers have linked soy to an early form of breast cancer

You may have heard that eating soy can protect you from developing breast cancer. There's research to say that's so! But, to quote a famous commentator: "Here's the rest of the story..."

In one significant study completed in 1996, researchers found that women who ate soy protein had an increased incidence of epithelial hyperplasia, an early form of malignancy. A year later, a chemical found in soy was shown to encourage breast cells to metastasize.

Does that mean soy causes some breast cancers? Well, again, no one can say for sure. But until scientists figure it all out, it's important for women to know about the potentially serious downsides.

And believe it or not, that's not all there is to know about soy...

You can get as much 'estrogen' eating soy protein as taking the birth control pill

You may have heard that soy contains beneficial substances called *isoflavones.* They're thought to improve symptoms associated with menopause. But isoflavones can also wreak havoc on your hormonal system.

Here's how...

One hundred grams of soy protein daily — the amount recommended by a national soy organization — provides the estrogenic equivalent of taking the birth control pill. If you're having symptoms of menopause, you'll likely reduce them with this hormonal boost from "soy estrogen."

But not so fast. You might be getting more than you bargain for...

In 1991, Japanese researchers found that as little as *two teaspoons of soy protein a day caused goiter and hyperthyroidism in some patients.* Isoflavones were believed to be the culprit.

Isoflavones are also thought to cause all

sorts of problems in infants. In fact, *an infant who is fed soy formula is getting the estrogenic equivalent of five birth control pills a day.* Some experts believe this excess estrogen can lead to thyroid problems, learning disabilities, and even premature sexual development.

That's a disturbing possibility, considering that nearly half of all bottle fed babies in the U.S. receive soy formula.

Recent research ties two or more servings a week of tofu with "accelerated brain aging"

One of the most shocking discoveries about soy came to light at the Third International Soy Symposium. On the last day of the symposium, one researcher presented his three-decade long study of Japanese-Americans living in Hawaii.

It showed a *significant statistical relationship between eating two or more servings of tofu a week and "accelerated brain aging."* Individuals who ate this amount of tofu in mid-life had lower cognitive function later in life and a greater incidence of Alzheimer's disease and dementia. Again, researchers believed isoflavones were the offenders.

The soy debate is far from over

The final verdict on soy might be years in coming. And there's no way to tell whether it will be "for" soy, "against" soy, or a "split decision." But there's one source where you can arm yourself with the knowledge you need to stay healthy…
Dr. Jonathan Wright.

In fact, Dr. Wright pioneered the work on an all-natural cancer fighter that's found in…of all places…mustard. Want the astonishing details? Keep reading…

CHAPTER TWELVE

'Mustard Effect' makes female cancers vanish

You knew vegetables can stave off cancer, but *cure* it?

Suddenly, a door just opened into a brand new world where miracles are possible even for cancer patients.

This stuff is so harmless, you could (and probably should) take some every day just to be on the safe side. *Yet it's so powerful*, even I was blown away when Dr. Wright delivered the breathtaking news...

A potentially deadly cancer has been wiped out in nearly 50% of cases by an extract from vegetables you eat for dinner

Thirty women with a deadly form of cervical cancer took part in this breakthrough research. And within just 12 weeks...

What's *your* heart-health worry?

- **HIGH CHOLESTEROL?** Ron's was well over 400, despite three years on a low-fat diet. Yet Dr. Wright's easy solution dropped his cholesterol 180 points…and his triglycerides plummeted by a staggering 540 points.

- **HARDENING OF THE ARTERIES?** Hernando's blockage was so advanced, he could barely hobble across a room! He said "I'm just waiting around for things to get bad enough so I can have my legs amputated." Yet thanks to Dr. Wright, he was walking "at least two miles, three times every week, without sitting down once!"

- **ANGINA?** John's vanished in just 10 days. His pain was so intense, that his doctor was urging *bypass surgery*, but Dr. Wright's natural solutions cleared it up in just over a week!

- **CONGESTIVE HEART FAILURE?** Mrs. Livingston's lungs were filled with fluid and she couldn't even sleep without being propped up. But Dr. Wright soon had her sleeping like a baby and feeling so strong, *she even started gardening again!*

Let Dr. Wright do the same for you and your loved ones. RSVP today to get your FREE BONUS *Library of Food & Vitamin Cures.*

Nearly half the women who ate the extract became totally cancer-free

The results shocked nearly every researcher who saw them, *except Dr. Wright.*

He had already been advising his patients to devour these veggies with gusto. They're commonly called *the mustard family* — mustard, broccoli, cauliflower, bok choy, cabbage and brussels sprouts all belong to the club.

They contain lots of good stuff, but their best secret is THE MIRACLE MOLECULE I3C

And ending cervical cancer is just the *start* of what I3C could do for us. It may also prove to be a long-sought key to combatting

- **Breast Cancer...**
- **Uterine Cancer...**
- **Ovarian Cancer...**

And every other kind of cancer that feeds on female sex hormones. Instead of attacking cancer cells, I3C reverses their ability to convert your estrogen mix from "bad" to "good."

Yes, there's 'bad' and 'good' estrogen! (This

has nothing to do with progesterone.) Dr. Wright is famous for having written about this long ago. And he confirmed they've got to be *balanced*, just like good and bad cholesterol, because...

- **Bad estrogen** feeds cancer in your breasts and sex organ tissues...

- **Good estrogen** inhibits this out-of-control cell growth...

It's a big reason why some women are more prone to cancer than others. It's the *type* of estrogen in your body that makes the difference. You'll find full details on how to check and correct your own estrogen balance in your FREE BONUS *Library of Food & Vitamin Cures*, so please do take the opportunity to RSVP now.

Next up... the one "Miracle Mineral" is revealed to you.

CHAPTER THIRTEEN

'Miracle Mineral' tackles everything from acne to arteriosclerosis!

If I told you a 'magic potion' existed that could:

- Make germ-infested water safe to drink...
- Take care of stubborn bladder infections...
- Help painful ovarian cysts disappear...
- Help hemorrhoids to vanish overnight...
- Even help dissolve built-up cholesterol...

You'd probably call me nuts. But such a super-cure actually exists — Dr. Wright recently revealed all the details to his *Nutrition & Healing* readers! And the best part is this: It's available in any corner drug store without a prescription... And for less than the cost of a cup of coffee! So what is this overlooked over-the-counter miracle healer? It's a special form of...ordinary *iodide*.

No, it's not the stuff you put on a cut —
but a closely related iodide compound called
SSKI that Dr. Wright has demonstrated is
actually one of nature's most miraculous
healers. He's found dozens of amazing uses
for it, and he'll pass along these secrets to
you in your FREE BONUS *Library of Food
& Vitamin Cures.* Lest you think I'm making
this up, let me explain how some of them
work right here...

SURPRISE 1:

Dr. Wright has a physician friend who drank contaminated water for 30 years, while ministering to African villagers...

...and the water was typically so foul, he
had to strain out the scum with a
cheesecloth! Yet he never got sick even once.
All he did was add a few drops of SSKI
iodide to the water a few minutes before he
drank it. Presto, it was drinkable.

SURPRISE 2:

Ever get sick after an airline flight?

Dr. Wright makes sure he doesn't. Before
he boards the airplane, he simply drinks
water mixed with a few drops of SSKI (he'll

explain what it is in your FREE Library).

The iodide rapidly travels to your nose, throat and sinuses. There it proceeds to zap hoards of bacteria and viruses floating around in that foul-smelling cabin air. Abracadabra, you're bug-proof!

SURPRISE 3:

Women know how painful bladder infections can be...

...and they always seem to flare up when your doctor isn't available. But Dr. Wright has shown his loved ones how to end the

Breast pain and cysts since she was a teenager... relieved in just 10 minutes

Jenny B. had painful cysts in her breasts since she was 17. They hurt so much, she said "I can't even sleep on my chest between periods. And if my husband even touches my breasts...well, it makes sex awfully tricky."

Dr. Wright found she had dozens of lumps in each breast, and swelling around the lumps. He knew it was caused by a deficiency — and problem all by themselves, with nothing more than an eyedropper and that trusty iodide bottle. According to Dr. Wright, it's close to 100% effective.

SURPRISE 4:

Ovarian cysts can be so agonizing that...

...many women gladly go under the knife just to be rid of them. Yet Dr. Wright has made them disappear for dozens of women, including his own daughter. No scalpels required, just that bottle of SSKI iodide! (Benign breast cysts vanish just as easily

gave her just two common minerals. Ten minutes after taking them, she could hardly believe the difference. "I'm better! I don't hurt as much and I think the swelling is less, I think even the lumpy areas are smaller."

Seven months later, she was even happier. "I haven't had any pain in two months now! All those lumps are a lot smaller and I think some of them are gone. I feel generally better all over!"

Full details about the treatment that healed her in your FREE BONUS Library. Return your exclusive Gift Certificate today.

with a similar treatment.)

SURPRISE 5:

Wake up to no more hemorrhoids

A colleague of Dr. Wright's has found that hemorrhoids really do vanish overnight when you simply mix iodide with a common vegetable oil and apply at bedtime. A similar technique can flatten enormous scars.

SURPRISE 6:

Dissolve cholesterol? Really?

Honest. As a student at Harvard, Dr. Wright never forgot a demonstration by famed chemistry professor Louis Feiser. Professor Feiser used iodide to dissolve all manner of oils, fats and waxes — and it so happens that cholesterol is a wax. He urged his students to remember this trick in their medical practices...

Dr. Wright did just that. And now he's using it in a breakthrough artery-clearing therapy. If you know anyone with arteriosclerosis, this could save his or her life.

How do I know?

Photographic proof, that's how. Doctors actually took photographs of patients' retinal

A note from Jonathan V. Wright, M.D.
"Just give your body a second chance and NOTHING IS HOPELESS!"

Dear Friend:

Patients often ask me how many of my treatments can work so much better, when big drug firms throw **billions of dollars** at trying to heal the same diseases.

Well, I certainly can't outspend them! But I do have the most powerful ally in all of medicine: **you and your amazing body.**

While drugs just work on symptoms, my therapies work with you and your body, to:

- **try to help your whole body** heal itself, so there isn't any pain to suppress...
- **work to eliminate the cause** of your suffering, so it won't bounce back when the drugs wear off...

And if that sounds like a tall order, surprise! I promise you, natural, nutritional medicine is not only far more effective "in the long run," but...

In the short run too. You may feel the first results within just a few days or even hours. Then keep improving until your old suffering is just a memory.

Believe me, whether your problem is as "chronic" as arthritis pain or as "incurable" as lupus or multiple sclerosis, I've found that very little is hopeless when your body's back in the fight.

The miracles we'll ever need are often **hidden inside you,** waiting to be released. Won't you give your body a second chance? Let me show you how.

Please do mail your no-risk GIFT CERTIFICATE today.

Your pioneering doctor,

Jonathan V. Wright, M.D.

arteries before and after a similar therapy. The published photos show a significant lessening of cholesterol-laden artery clogging.

CAUTION: Do not try these before reading Dr. Wright's detailed instructions.

SSKI iodide has enormous potential benefits, but you do need to know how to avoid the hazards. Please wait until you receive your FREE BONUS Library. He'll give you instructions for all the tricks above and explain the fascinating biochemistry that makes it work so wonderfully. But there's more...

SURPRISES 7, 8 AND 9:

Eliminate life's most embarrassing complaints

You can also zap unsightly new acne zits in 24-48 hours, cure stubborn cases of toenail fungus, wipe out the cause of flatulence...and more, all with that one little SSKI bottle. So isn't it time you sent for your own FREE BONUS *Library of Food & Vitamin Cures?* An RSVP Gift Certificate came with your book (and there are others at the back of this book).

CHAPTER FOURTEEN

Why wait in the pain-wracked past? Step into your fabulous future... FREE!

As you've seen, thanks to Dr. Jonathan V. Wright, medicine's future is already here and working true miracles. Tens of thousands of readers of Dr. Wright's *Nutrition & Healing* have already felt the miraculous effects of his new kind of medicine...

But you may have to wait for decades unless you act now

Awesome as they are, Dr. Wright's discoveries will not be mainstreamed if the drug establishment has its way. Bear in mind these vested interests could lose hundreds of billions of dollars if his amazingly cheap and simple solutions replaced costly drugs. And unthinkable as it sounds...

Drug interests have officially declared war on vitamins

Imagine a world where safe nutritional supplements are locked away like narcotics. Where it's even illegal to buy vitamin pills without begging for a doctor's prescription. This isn't paranoia...

It's already happening all across Europe

The European Parliament recently passed a "Directive on Dietary Supplements." Under this directive, which became law in 2005, certain vitamins and minerals are classified as drugs. Except for certain "approved" supplements that don't appear on the positive list, all other supplements will be banned from over-the-counter sale.

This isn't just an inconvenience, it's premeditated murder! For example...

In Chapter Five, you read how Dr. Wright's selenium discovery could save millions of men from prostate cancer...

Yet under the new directive, this essential mineral will be swept off the shelves and locked away as a dangerous prescription drug. The European Parliament doesn't think you can be trusted with it. And Europe's just the testing ground. The intent is for this model to be adopted everywhere...

Don't think it can't happen here

Drug interests have already worked relentlessly to pull cholesterol-lowering yeast supplements from the market. They've succeeded in banning the essential amino acid L-Tryptophan. They're conspiring with the FDA to take all-natural bioidentical hormones away from you. And these are just three examples of why you won't get Dr. Wright's breakthroughs unless you demand them...

So do it today — claim your FREE BONUS *Library of Food & Vitamin Cures* right now

And free the incredibly healthy human being that's locked up inside of you! To claim your FREE *Library of Food & Vitamin Cures,* just use the "Gift Certificate" enclosed with this book and mail it in the enclosed postage-free envelope. You'll get all 8 lifesaving, life-giving volumes, plus...

An unbeatable, money saving deal on today's most honored alternative health newsletter

When Dr. Wright's colleagues honored him with The Linus Pauling Award, they gave special praise to his cutting-edge health advisory, *Nutrition & Healing*.

This is the only alternative health newsletter I know of that counts so many doctors among its subscribers. Because it's the real stuff. The first place where you'll learn what new breakthroughs are coming down the road from natural medicine's living legend.

Everything's reported in crystal-clear language, telling you exactly how to go out and do it. But *Nutrition & Healing* gives you all the science too. So if your doctor ever questions any remedy you read about here, just pull out your newsletter and produce the proof. Any truly objective doctor can't help being impressed with the quality of Dr. Wright's research. (Warning: your doctor may ask to keep the issue!)

No other newsletter of its kind is more respected by natural physicians and actually

Read this if you're still wondering whether Dr. Wright's breakthroughs can help you and your loved ones

Dear Dr. Wright,

I just wanted to write and *thank you for the wonderful year I have just had.* I have not had one migraine since I left your office. This might come as a shock, but I'm not writing this letter about my migraine. When I was in your office, I read a few issues of your newsletter, *Nutrition & Healing*. I ended up subscribing — and applying that information to some problems at home.

You see, my father has Alzheimer's disease. A year ago, he did not know any of us and had terrible hallucinations. I did a little research in your newsletter and found all the information I needed. I ordered the products that you recommended and I immediately started seeing improvement.

Even my physician is surprised with the progress — maybe he'll even apply some of this knowledge to his practice. My father now knows who his family is and can even play cards again, one of his passions.

Every condition that comes up in our household, from my mother's arthritis, which by the way is not bothering her anymore, to my husband's sinus and ear infections. According to his ear specialist, my husband has been able to avoid ear surgery.

All of this has been possible through your newsletter, *Nutrition & Healing*. Between the case study, the nutrient of the month and the interviews, everything I needed was there.

We can never repay you for the happiness that has been possible from your newsletter, but the least we could do is thank you. Please keep up the good work!

In Good Health,

Velda

Velda K., Phoenix, AZ

used by them to heal their own patients. And no other newsletter will do more to heal you...

Because this isn't just 'health news.' *Each issue is like a complete instruction book for healing yourself.* Complete with dosages, sources for the hard-to-find nutrients Dr. Wright recommends, and all the pros and cons that you (and your doctor!) need to make an informed decision.

The enclosed "Gift Certificate" saves you $25 on your risk-free subscription to Dr. Wright's *Nutrition & Healing.* And brings you Dr. Wright's complete library for reversing nearly a hundred "incurable" conditions, including his most acclaimed formulas and programs, FREE.

There's no obligation to continue your subscription unless you're thrilled with your first issue. If you're not, just say the word, and we'll send you a full pro-rated refund. And you can keep your FREE BONUS GIFTS.

Just promise me you'll start using your FREE BONUS GIFTS as soon as you get them...

And as soon as you do, I promise, you'll feel a little stronger every morning, feel a little less pain every evening, until one fine day, you wake up and realize…

'I don't need to risk my life to FEEL FABULOUS!'

I guarantee your day will arrive very soon. Or just tell us and we'll send you a prompt refund on all unmailed issues. You'll KEEP YOUR FREE BONUS GIFTS no matter what.

Fair enough? So do let me hear from you now.

Let Dr. Wright push the envelope of what's possible for you…

And step into his amazing new world where health miracles are commonplace…

Make it happen today! RSVP right now.

Here's to the dawn of a bright new day in your health,

Matthew Simons

Matthew Simons
Publisher

P.S. FAST-REPLY GIFT! Respond within 11 days, and I'll rush you Dr. Wright's brand-new report, The Miracle Mineral. Find out how he's ending everything from acne to arteriosclerosis ...clearing up everything from hemorrhoids to ovarian cysts... even banishing drug-resistant disease germs...all with one little "magic bottle." Don't wait another day to claim this lifesaving FREE BONUS!

P.P.S. As an added bonus, if you respond within the next five days, you'll get a FREE 8th volume in your *Library of Food & Vitamin Cures:* Dr. Wright's New Secrets for Healing Your 'Incurable' Hurts. You'll get Dr. Wright's best time-tested natural remedies for asthma, MS, wound healing, chronic pain, gallbladder pain, hay fever, vision loss and so much more. Supplies are limited...RSVP now.

Your FREE BONUS 8-VOLUME Library of Food & Vitamin Cures

A message to you from Dr. Jonathan Wright...

"These new natural remedies are your birthright as a human being..."

So please accept my complete new *Library of Food & Vitamin Cures* FREE. Reply now for all 8 volumes free with your subscription to *Nutrition & Healing*

VOLUME 1:

Dr. Wright's New Secrets for Reading Your Body Like A Book

Dr. Wright's
New Secrets
for
**Reading
Your Body
Like
A Book**

Look in the mirror tonight and you'll see secret clues all over your body. They're your keys to wiping out ailments that puzzled you for years.

Varicose veins…broken fingernails… "skin tags" on your neck or under your arms…forehead wrinkles…bursitis…they're often just the "tip of the iceberg" for hidden problems that cause heart disease, crippling arthritis, senility, premature aging and more. Your remedy could be as simple as one or two vitamins and minerals. Learn this secret language…

Even if you're in the late stages of an "incurable" condition, it's not too late to turn your health around. 100 lupus patients were cured by just one of these new natural breakthroughs, and there's fantastic news too about chronic fatigue, memory loss and much more…

VOLUME 2:

Dr. Wright's New Secrets for Repairing Your Heart & Arteries

Dr. Wright's
New Secrets
for
**Repairing
Your Heart
& Arteries**

Drop your cholesterol 134 points without drugs or deprivation. Find out how David did it. (Dr. Wright added food to his diet!) Far healthier than statin drugs and increases your energy too…

Slashes edema, lung congestion,

shortness of breath and palpitations. In a new study, 80% of heart patients who tried it got better! So how come no one's told you about the nutrient *OPC?* Here's your #1 source…

If your blood pressure's high, you can take drugs. But why trade stroke-risk for weakness or even impotence? Dr. Wright's patients often drop it to normal from as high as 170 and throw out their drugs. It's not hard — one common nutrient alone can reduce systolic pressure by 18 points. Do a little more and it can drop 20, 30, even 40 points…

Angina pain plummets in 77% of patients. Time after time, this amazing natural substance has brought Dr. Wright's cardiac patients back from the brink of death to a healthy, full life. Low levels in your blood are now linked to hardened arteries, high cholesterol, high triglycerides, high blood pressure and even obesity. How to check your levels and where to get it…

Cardiomyopathy normally kills 3/4 of its victims within two years of their first attack. But now you can lift the death sentence. 60% of those who supplemented with just one nutrient were alive and kicking even five years later. Given that we all need it, isn't this a no-brainer?

VOLUME 3:

Dr. Wright's New Secrets for Success with Arthritis

The 100% Solution. Folks with inflammatory arthritis must be the most "patient patients" in the world — so many new drugs, so few results! But Dr. Wright has discovered an easy, painless, side-effect-free nutrition program that does what no drug can claim. It's produced results for nearly all of the *hundreds* of patients who've tried it. For some, it reduces the swelling and pain. For others, all of it goes away. Shouldn't you at least know about it?

Which joint pain supplements really work? Dr. Wright's research shows that the best are among the cheapest. None are patented, proprietary or even trendy, but put them together and the effect can be miraculous. Learn the formula and put away the Prednisone® and aspirin for good.

The $10 cure for pain and swelling of osteoarthritis. Dr. Wright's been using it for more than 25 years. Offers astonishing relief to the large majority of his patients. Give it just three weeks and start feeling the pain melt away. A vitamin that costs all of $10 a bottle…

If wear and tear cause arthritis, how come so many long-distance runners never get it, but their sedentary friends do? Look no further than the food you eat. One type of food in particular can switch it on and off with uncanny precision. Avoid a few vegetables and your "worn out" joints could soon feel like new again.

VOLUME 4:

Dr. Wright's New Secrets for Potency, Vitality & Prostate Health

Dr. Wright's
New Secrets
for
**Potency,
Vitality &
Prostate
Health**

The #1 forbidden topic that every man *must* know about. What is it that turns strong, healthy men into doddering, mentally dull old codgers? It's not Father Time, but a simple decline in *testosterone!* Just raising the levels can turn a man's sex life around. Reverse years of declining strength. *Plus* reduce your risk of heart disease, make your joints hurt less, make your memory sharper…and yes, even protect you from prostate disease. Learn the truth about *natural* testosterone…

"But isn't testosterone dangerous?"

No, *the stuff in all the scare stories isn't testosterone at all.*

Toxic "anabolic steroids" are actually synthetic imitations, created by drug companies because you can't patent natural testosterone. That's the same reason you'll see so many ads for Viagra® and none for natural testosterone therapy.

Yet the latter can be far safer…

"So where do I get it?"

Real, natural testosterone is not on the shelves of many pharmacies. You must know who to ask and what to ask for. Let Dr. Wright give you complete details about where to find it and how to get a prescription, including phone and fax numbers. This may be the only place you'll ever find this information…

What drug companies don't want me to know is that, thanks to a biochemical breakthrough, we now can make identical-to-nature testosterone from *plants.*

It's very safe if administered properly.

Unlike Viagra®, it restores your libido. And unlike hi-tech, patented products like Androderm®, true-to-nature testosterone isn't terribly expensive...

VOLUME 5:

Dr. Wright's New Secrets Every Woman Needs to Know

The "hormone replacement therapy" prescribed by most doctors does not replace your natural hormone balance. In fact, it fills you with horse hormones! But you've got a natural alternative that's more effective and safer too. Maybe you've heard of natural hormone therapy, *but did you know Dr. Wright introduced it?*

Thousands of his patients have been using it safely for nearly 20 years. Let him tell you the little-known facts that every woman needs to know about the real thing...

Instead of just halting bone loss, wouldn't it be great to *increase* your bone density? Now it's possible, even if you're well past age 60. And this is just one benefit of Dr. Wright's natural hormone therapy. Find out how to get it in your area...

If you think fibroids are painful, wait until you try surgery! But Dr. Wright has a natural solution that can save you from the scalpel. In an open study, this herbal formula improved fibroids or totally normalized things — for well over half of all premenopausal women. How to get it...

The longevity hormone. Your adrenal glands produce about 70 different hormones. This one's the most abundant, but your doctor probably hasn't even mentioned it! After age 30, a woman's production can plummet. Low levels are found in women with rheumatoid arthritis, lupus, type 1 diabetes, and a whole range of cancers. Every woman over age 60 should be sure she's making enough of it. How to get tested and get the therapy...

VOLUME 6:

Dr. Wright's New Secrets — The Astonishing Eggplant Cure for Cancer

Dr. Wright's
New Secrets
The Astonishing Eggplant Cure for Cancer

Cancer cure with a 100% success rate. And, amazingly, this breakthrough treatment is a form of an eggplant extract. Learn the facts about this cancer-killing miracle...

Can even be used cosmetically — to eradicate age spots, sun spots and "pre-cancers" like actinic keratoses. It's non-invasive, nontoxic and so easy to use you can do it at home…

More than 80,000 patients over the past 26 years have used this extract to treat non-melanoma skin cancer. Microscopic analysis consistently shows death of *all* cancer cells. Better yet, *no cancer has ever returned*…

The only way to learn about this no-fail cure… you would never have heard about this astounding cancer treatment if not for Dr. Jonathan Wright. You see, it threatens the pocketbooks of pharmaceutical firms, dermatology clinics and plastic surgeons…

VOLUME 7:

The Miracle Mineral

RSVP in 11 days to get this astonishing new report FREE!

Imagine ending *dozens* of serious health threats with just a few drops of one common mineral. Thanks to Dr. Wright, it's not science fiction anymore! Let him show you how it can:

Wipe out the deadliest germs without

antibiotics! Cures nearly 100% of bladder infections. Protects you from respiratory diseases in germ laden "airplane air." A physician friend of Dr. Wright's used it to make disease-infested water safe to drink. *In 30 years, traveling all over Africa, he never got sick even once.*

Make painful hemorrhoids vanish *overnight.* Cause painful ovarian cysts and breast cysts to *disappear* without surgery. Even end embarrassing *acne* in 24-48 hours and...

Yes, even reverse arteriosclerosis. Photographs have documented how supplements containing this mineral visibly reduce arteriosclerotic clogging of arteries. It literally *dissolves* waxy cholesterol deposits. And these are just a *few* of the many miracles you can perform with it. Learn them all!

VOLUME 8:

Dr. Wright's New Secrets for Healing Your 'Incurable' Hurts.

FREE FASTER Reply Bonus — Get it FREE by responding in the next 5 days!

Asthma's new nonsteroid solution.

One vitamin and one mineral. That's it! Put them together and watch them stop even an acute asthma attack with dazzling speed...

Best news in years about MS. A brand-new, all-natural skin patch could do for MS victims what insulin shots did for diabetics. In the latest research, it helped patients move their limbs for the first time in years, stand, walk, even drive cars. Find out how to get it...

Dozens more nutritional miracles including enzymes that heal cuts and bruises faster... vitamin "cocktail" that erased chronic pain in 30 seconds... the painless nutritional program that's making 99% of gallbladder surgery unnecessary... and a whole lot more.

Over 60% of the miseries that you thought were incurable have now been linked to a single, secret culprit. Dr. Wright has long said we could cut our health problems in half simply by detecting our secret food sensitivities. Now a major corporate study proves he's right on the money! Learn the technique and watch hay fever, bronchitis, back pain, colitis, ulcers and even hyperactivity *disappear*...

The most common type of age-related vision loss is totally unnecessary in 70% of all cases. It's much the same story with hearing loss. New studies link the latter to a lack of just two common vitamins. And now both can be prevented, halted and even *reversed* with incredible ease.

Get your FREE
Library of Food &
Vitamin Cures today!

Dr. Wright's New Secrets for **Reading Your Body Like A Book**	Dr. Wright's New Secrets for **Repairing Your Heart & Arteries**	Dr. Wright's New Secrets for **Success with Arthritis**	Dr. Wright's New Secrets for **Potency, Vitality & Prostate Health**	Dr. Wright's New Secrets **Every Woman Needs to Know**	Dr. Wright's New Secrets **The Astonishing Eggplant Cure for Cancer**

Reply in 11 days and receive one more FREE gift!

Get another FREE bonus if you reply in 5 days!

The Miracle Mineral

Dr. Wright's New Secrets for **Healing Your 'Incurable' Hurts**

LIFETIME GUARANTEE:

At any time, for any reason—if you're not satisfied with Dr. Wright's NUTRITION & HEALING, just drop us a note and we'll send you a refund for all unmailed issues right away. No questions asked and, of course, KEEP YOUR FREE GIFTS.

Do it now! Cut out this RSVP GIFT CERTIFICATE and mail it today!

☐ **YES, DR. WRIGHT!** Rush me my FREE Library of Food & Vitamin Cures and enter my risk-free subscription now.

   ☐ **SAVE $25. Receive 6 FREE GIFTS!** 1 year (12 issues) for only $49. (49AR)(021)

   ☐ **FAST REPLY BONUS! 7 FREE GIFTS!** I'm responding in 11 days. Send my FREE BONUS, *The Miracle Mineral*.

   ☐ **FASTER REPLY BONUS! 8 FREE GIFTS IN ALL!** I'm responding in 5 days — so I get another FREE bonus.

Method of Payment:

☐ Check or money order made out to Dr. Wright's NUTRITION & HEALING. (Maryland residents please add 6% sales tax.)

Charge my credit card: ☐ VISA ☐ MC ☐ AMEX ☐ Discover

_____

Card Number   Exp. Date

_____

Name

_____

Signature

_____

Address

_____

City/State/Zip Code

_____

Phone Number (in case we have a question about your order)

_____

E-mail (If you wish to receive our Dr. Wright's FREE Health eTips service. We never share your email address)

By paying by credit card, you are selecting our Preferred Subscriber Benefit. This guarantees you receive continuous service and never miss one of Dr. Wright's lifesaving breakthroughs. After your initial subscription term is complete, your credit card will be billed our lowest annual rate of $49. This convenient service guarantees your subscription continues as long as you want and you always receive our lowest annual rate. There is no obligation; you can still cancel at *any time* to get a full refund on all your unmailed issues.

Mail to: Nutrition & Healing, Order Processing Center P.O. Box 925, Frederick, MD 21705-9913   **DNHDL801**

DNH0810-RPLY

CIR-P   T1/12

Get your FREE *Library of Food & Vitamin Cures* today!

Dr. Wright's New Secrets for **Reading Your Body Like A Book**

Dr. Wright's New Secrets for **Repairing Your Heart & Arteries**

Dr. Wright's New Secrets for **Success with Arthritis**

Dr. Wright's New Secrets for **Potency, Vitality & Prostate Health**

Dr. Wright's New Secrets **Every Woman Needs to Know**

Dr. Wright's New Secrets **The Astonishing Eggplant Cure for Cancer**

Reply in 11 days and receive one more FREE gift!

Get another FREE bonus if you reply in 5 days!

The Miracle Mineral

Dr. Wright's New Secrets for **Healing Your 'Incurable' Hurts**

LIFETIME GUARANTEE:

At any time, for any reason—if you're not satisfied with Dr. Wright's NUTRITION & HEALING, just drop us a note and we'll send you a refund for all unmailed issues right away. No questions asked and, of course, KEEP YOUR FREE GIFTS.

Do it now! Cut out this RSVP GIFT CERTIFICATE and mail it today!

☐ **YES, DR. WRIGHT!** Rush me my FREE Library of Food & Vitamin Cures and enter my risk-free subscription now.

  ☐ **SAVE $25. Receive 6 FREE GIFTS!** 1 year (12 issues) for only $49. (49AR)(021)

  ☐ **FAST REPLY BONUS! 7 FREE GIFTS!** I'm responding in 11 days. Send my FREE BONUS, *The Miracle Mineral*.

  ☐ **FASTER REPLY BONUS! 8 FREE GIFTS IN ALL!** I'm responding in 5 days — so I get another FREE bonus.

Method of Payment:

☐ Check or money order made out to Dr. Wright's NUTRITION & HEALING. (Maryland residents please add 6% sales tax.)

Charge my credit card: ☐ VISA   ☐ MC   ☐ AMEX   ☐ Discover

Card Number _____ Exp. Date _____

Name _____

Signature _____

Address _____

City/State/Zip Code _____

Phone Number (in case we have a question about your order) _____

E-mail (If you wish to receive our Dr. Wright's FREE Health eTips service. We never share your email address) _____

By paying by credit card, you are selecting our Preferred Subscriber Benefit. This guarantees you receive continuous service and never miss one of Dr. Wright's lifesaving breakthroughs. After your initial subscription term is complete, your credit card will be billed our lowest annual rate of $49. This convenient service guarantees your subscription continues as long as you want and you always receive our lowest annual rate. There is no obligation; you can still cancel at *any time* to get a full refund on all your unmailed issues.

Mail to: Nutrition & Healing, Order Processing Center
P.O. Box 925, Frederick, MD 21705-9913 | DNHDL801 |

DNH0810-RPLY

CIR-P   T1/12

Get your FREE *Library of Food & Vitamin Cures* today!

Dr. Wright's New Secrets for Reading Your Body Like A Book

Dr. Wright's New Secrets for Repairing Your Heart & Arteries

Dr. Wright's New Secrets for Success with Arthritis

Dr. Wright's New Secrets for Potency, Vitality & Prostate Health

Dr. Wright's New Secrets Every Woman Needs to Know

Dr. Wright's New Secrets The Astonishing Eggplant Cure for Cancer

Reply in 11 days and receive one more FREE gift!

The Miracle Mineral

Get another FREE bonus if you reply in 5 days!

Dr. Wright's New Secrets for Healing Your 'Incurable' Hurts

LIFETIME GUARANTEE:

At any time, for any reason—if you're not satisfied with Dr. Wright's NUTRITION & HEALING, just drop us a note and we'll send you a refund for all unmailed issues right away. No questions asked and, of course, KEEP YOUR FREE GIFTS.

Do it now! Cut out this RSVP GIFT CERTIFICATE and mail it today!

Get your FREE *Library of Food & Vitamin Cures* today!

Dr. Wright's New Secrets for **Reading Your Body Like A Book**

Dr. Wright's New Secrets for **Repairing Your Heart & Arteries**

Dr. Wright's New Secrets for **Success with Arthritis**

Dr. Wright's New Secrets for **Potency, Vitality & Prostate Health**

Dr. Wright's New Secrets **Every Woman Needs to Know**

Dr. Wright's New Secrets **The Astonishing Eggplant Cure for Cancer**

Reply in 11 days and receive one more FREE gift!

Get another FREE bonus if you reply in 5 days!

The Miracle Mineral

Dr. Wright's New Secrets for **Healing Your 'Incurable' Hurts**

LIFETIME GUARANTEE:

At any time, for any reason—if you're not satisfied with Dr. Wright's NUTRITION & HEALING, just drop us a note and we'll send you a refund for all unmailed issues right away. No questions asked and, of course, KEEP YOUR FREE GIFTS.

DNH0810-RPLY

Do it now! Cut out this RSVP GIFT CERTIFICATE and mail it today!

☐ **YES, DR. WRIGHT!** Rush me my FREE Library of Food & Vitamin Cures and enter my risk-free subscription now.

  ☐ **SAVE $25. Receive 6 FREE GIFTS!** 1 year (12 issues) for only $49. (49AR)(021)

  ☐ **FAST REPLY BONUS! 7 FREE GIFTS!** I'm responding in 11 days. Send my FREE BONUS, *The Miracle Mineral*.

  ☐ **FASTER REPLY BONUS! 8 FREE GIFTS IN ALL!** I'm responding in 5 days — so I get another FREE bonus.

Method of Payment:

☐ Check or money order made out to Dr. Wright's NUTRITION & HEALING. (Maryland residents please add 6% sales tax.)

Charge my credit card: ☐ VISA ☐ MC ☐ AMEX ☐ Discover

_____
Card Number   Exp. Date

_____
Name

_____
Signature

_____
Address

_____
City/State/Zip Code

_____
Phone Number (in case we have a question about your order)

_____
E-mail (If you wish to receive our Dr. Wright's FREE Health eTips service. We never share your email address)

By paying by credit card, you are selecting our Preferred Subscriber Benefit. This guarantees you receive continuous service and never miss one of Dr. Wright's lifesaving breakthroughs. After your initial subscription term is complete, your credit card will be billed our lowest annual rate of $49. This convenient service guarantees your subscription continues as long as you want and you always receive our lowest annual rate. There is no obligation; you can still cancel at *any time* to get a full refund on all your unmailed issues.

Mail to: Nutrition & Healing, Order Processing Center
P.O. Box 925, Frederick, MD 21705-9913   **DNHDL801**

T1/12

CIR-P

Get your FREE *Library of Food & Vitamin Cures* today!

Dr. Wright's New Secrets for **Reading Your Body Like A Book**

Dr. Wright's New Secrets for **Repairing Your Heart & Arteries**

Dr. Wright's New Secrets for **Success with Arthritis**

Dr. Wright's New Secrets for **Potency, Vitality & Prostate Health**

Dr. Wright's New Secrets **Every Woman Needs to Know**

Dr. Wright's New Secrets **The Astonishing Eggplant Cure for Cancer**

Reply in 11 days and receive one more FREE gift!

Get another FREE bonus if you reply in 5 days!

The Miracle Mineral

Dr. Wright's New Secrets for **Healing Your 'Incurable' Hurts**

LIFETIME GUARANTEE:

At any time, for any reason—if you're not satisfied with Dr. Wright's NUTRITION & HEALING, just drop us a note and we'll send you a refund for all unmailed issues right away. No questions asked and, of course, KEEP YOUR FREE GIFTS.

He remembered confessing once to a friend, Tommy Cantin, in the seventh grade that he was not allowed to answer the telephone. Tommy had stared at him in disbelief, as if he were a creature from an alien planet. Everybody in America answers the phone, Tommy had said. *Not me,* he had answered. But he was sixteen now—that made a difference.

He went to the bathroom. Closed the door and flushed the toilet, watching the swirling water, the sound obliterating the ringing of the phone. He had used this ploy before.

Emerging from the bathroom, he swore softly—"son of a bitch"—as the phone continued to ring. He had lost count. Must be up to twenty-nine, thirty by now. Still going strong, the sound ominous and threatening.

The record for the afternoon was eighteen rings last year. This was absurd. Thirty-eight? Thirty-nine?

Maybe it was an emergency.

His father injured at work. Or his mother in an accident.

An urgency now in the ringing, filling the rooms, filling his ears, vibrating throughout his body.

He had to stop this crazy ringing.

But he knew the rule. His father's rule: *Do not pick up the phone. Let your mother or me answer it. If it's for you, I will hand it over. Alone in the house, you do not answer.*

Emergency or not, he had to stop the ringing.